Eft

Tapping

An Effective Tapping Solution To Build Self-Confidence

(Transformation Through Emotional Freedom Therapy Tapping)

Jeffrey Crocker

Published By **Bella Frost**

Jeffrey Crocker

All Rights Reserved

Eft Tapping: An Effective Tapping Solution To Build Self-Confidence (Transformation Through Emotional Freedom Therapy Tapping)

ISBN   978-1-77485-690-1

No part of this guidebook shall be reproduced in any form without permission in writing from the publisher except in the case of brief quotations embodied in critical articles or reviews.

Legal & Disclaimer

TABLE OF CONTENTS

Chapter 1: The Making Maker

EFT is known as the Emotional Freedom Technique and emotional treatment that originates out of the Chinese Meridian system.

It's similar to acupuncture but we don't employ needles. Instead, we employ a simple two-pronged method that uses the mental part of it to be able to sense your emotions and then fix the issue by stimulating specific meridian points in the body by tapping the points with our fingers.

Our bodies are energy systems, and possess distinct electrical characteristics. This is something we learn early in the classroom or, at the very least, we ought to be taught about this.

For instance, if you walk with your feet bare on carpet, if your fingertip comes into contact with something, you can feel the impact.

What is it that makes EFT as well as The Faster Tapping Method similar or different? First of all, both require tapping on Meridian points.

They are both painless to use, so there is no need to be concerned about any anxiety. There is no need to poke ourselves with needles like you do with the acupuncture treatment.

Through both approaches, it can get straight to the root of the issues, and explains the reasons why there is a natural resistance from the majority of people leaving behind their old patterns and habits.

It might be shocking for the majority of people because they aren't aware of the reason for this or that. They aren't aware of the issue, or admit that they are suffering from an issue.

Another major difference is that both have excellent percentages of success. Many have stated that EFT has proven to be effective and has long-lasting results.

In this day and age that is full of fast fixes as well as magical pills, people seek tangible outcomes. What I like most about both of them is that they assist many people who are struggling to take charge of the healing process themselves.

A lot of people don't have the time or funds to go to an accredited EFT practitioner for emotional problems. The best part about the Faster Tapping Method is that users can apply this method anytime.

We'll now look at the many benefits of EFT and the Quicker Tapping Technique. Classic EFT believes that every emotional stress results from a disturbance of the body's energy system.

In traditional EFT the belief is that memory can be a factor, but they are not the reason behind negative emotions. The main cause is change in the emotional charge. If the energy pattern system is disturbed it causes physical and emotional stress.

A few years ago, when I first discovered the traditional EFT and began to use the technique and started to see positive improvements in my life. I'm a firm believer that the reasons we experience problems is due to the body's energetic system that is being disturbed.

Tapping on the meridian points of your body, it eliminates the blockage by restoring the movement of your energy. After having studied and using the technique, it seemed like it could not get better but it did when you apply the Faster tapping method (More on the method later).

Tapping is a great option for no matter what your experience or location or what you've been through previously. Through the Faster Tapping Method it will target the mind and body system through electrical impulses which travel through the Meridian System.

What exactly does Tapping help solve? Thanks to modern science, we've been able to find out some amazing results with tapping. The following are the results:

It can cause damage to the neuronal connections that connect the brain and body.

• Reprogram your brain.

Retrains and rewires neural pathways.

* The brain is able to change its code.

Changes our mood that will change our daily activities.

The main difference between the two techniques is that of Psychological Reversal. Our subconscious mind's main goal as humans is to ensure our safety.

One way that the subconscious mind performs this involves refusing change. When we are children, we form certain patterns of thinking. The first thing we learn is to live life with a cautious attitude and to remain safe in all that we do. At an early age, we've been taught to be resistant to changes.

The best part is that since we're in direct contact with your subconscious mind, and of its sources, if there's any fear or resistance , we should tap it and say a few affirmations.

For instance, "It's safe to let go of it." "I got through that incident and I'm in a safe place." "It's nothing of a problem." "And it's fine." "Be calm, let go."

Through affirming and reassuring words, we can be capable of changing our mood instantly.

After you've discovered how the Faster Tapping Method is different.

Let's look at how the process of applying the method works.

Chapter 2: The First Tapping Session

EFT is based on a few fundamental concepts that are universally recognized as a valid method of practice. these principles form the basis to this program.

While EFT is often disregarded as a therapy or success tool However, it has proven successful in the attainment of major life goals, the elimination of unpleasant and negative emotions, and also reduces and improves the physical ailments.

Tapping Locations & Technique:

There are two aspects of practicing EFT.

The first component that is EFT is the body points on your body which you tap and the sequence in which you tap the points in.

The second step is to define, frame and tackle the issue you're trying to solve.

Part 1: Tapping

The right points to tap at the appropriate time isn't considered to be crucial, but the power that EFT offers is not to be underestimated. When you properly apply the EFT pressure points you'll swiftly build a sense and control in your life.

Although EFT is a comfortable and universal practice the process of tapping itself is very precise with respect to meridians. It takes only just a few minutes to master but understanding the fundamentals of EFT can lead to an enjoyable experience.

Once you've got the hang of it, each round should take about one minute. A successful session will take only seven rounds.

Your fingers are the king of TAPPING:

Your fingertips provide you with powerful access to meridians that run through the entire body. They do not just let you access the meridians that are connected to the points you're tapping but they also allow you to unlock the meridians within which connect to your fingers. This combination creates a powerful influence inside your body, which alters and lets out even the most destructive negative feelings in your life.

Classic EFT utilizes the the index finger with the tips of your middle finger for tapping specific points in the body. It is possible to utilize one hand to tap on both sides of your body to get amazing results. It's important to note that you must remove all jewelry on your neck, eyes or head in order to let your body be free of energy. This includes watches, glasses, necklaces as well as bracelets. You can even remove your cap or hat.

If you'd like the hands to be rotated between each round to create a balanced effect. If you decide to tap two hands simultaneously then use your hands in alternate way rather than simultaneously. That is, tap 14 times at a time instead of two simultaneous taps with seven repeated taps.

While it's not essential to tap seven times for each point it's highly beneficial to take a full breath each time you tap.

The Tapping Points

There are 10 essential elements inside EFT. They are easy to locate and simple to remember. They will be listed below together with abbreviations to make the process simple to follow.

Point 1 Your skull's top (TH)

The location of this is at the the top of your skull.

Second point: the tip of your eyebrow(EB)

This position is situated close to the edges of your eyebrow, right above the nose. It is right next to your third eye.

3. The exterior part of your eye. (SE)

At the edges of the bone surrounding the eye is where this spot is located. The exact location is just to the left of the edge of your eye. On the bone, move straight towards the middle, or directly in line with your pupil. You can also do this by taking make a slightly.

Fourth Point: Under Your Eye (UE)

This point is situated approximately an inch beneath your pupils.

Fiveth point: directly beneath your nose (UN)

Directly below your nose and over your lower lip, this area is easy to spot.

6. Directly over the chin. (Ch)

This location is as easy as the previous. It's located just below the 5th point. It's located below the lower lip and just above the chin.

Seventh point: the collar bone. (CB)

The point is at the point where your sternum your collarbone and your first rib connect. This is a crucial point to the field of acupuncture, also known as K27. To locate this point locate mid-portion of the breastbone. (This is the place where a tie would go in the case of a man wearing tie.) If you notice the small cut on your chest.

When you have found it then move your finger downwards one inch, and then move it to the opposite side for a quarter of an inch.

Point 8: On the left side of the ribs (UA)

Directly on the side of your body in mid-ribs. this area is situated exactly parallel to the man's nipple or the middle of a woman's bra strap. If you're having difficulty then move about four inches beneath your armpit.

Point 9 in the center the wrist. (WR)

The final point is just at the center of wrists.

Point 10 10. It is the Karate Chop (KC)

The Karate Chop is positioned in the middle of the outside hand, which is in the opposite direction to the thumb. It's been cleverly designated as the Karate Chop point, making it easy to locate. If you're struggling to locate the point, consider the middle of the area where your wrist and hand meet and the point where your hand changes into your pinkie fingers.

For a better graphic representation, check out an example of tapping solutions that will give an excellent visual representation of all the points of EFT:

https://www.youtube.com/watch?v=pAclBdj20ZU

The TAPPING ORDER FOR EFT:

Point 10 (KC) (KC), point 2 (EB) Point 3 (SE) (SE), point 4, (UE) Point 5 (UN)

Point 6 (CH) Point 7 (CB) Point 8 (UA) point 9 (WR) followed by one point (TH).

Part II: how to recognize the root of your challenges.

The second part is the engine part of part 2 of the EFT system.

Once you've mastered the tapping points that are part of EFT It's time to turn our attention towards how you talk about and think about your emotional and mental situation while performing an EFT exercise. Here, you'll be taught the best way to frame your subject and the fundamentals of EFT and how to perform the first EFT exercise.

This method was first modeled by and subsequently uncovered through Gary Craig. This type is used and used in self-help for over 100 years.

A Simple Tapping Recipe: Five Steps to Relieve Stress

These five steps are easy to grasp and once you have grasped the idea, EFT will be a easy task to master every day.

Step 1: Determine your current situation.

Most of the time, you move through your life knowing that you're anxious and stressed. While identifying your emotions is the first step, it's crucial to determine the reason you are feeling anxious and deal with the issue.

While it's fine and beneficial to get rid of general issues with EFT however, it's highly efficient to deal with one problem at a given time, then move onto the next one after having solved the first issue.

If, for instance, you're feeling stressed about the whole relationship, it could be better to concentrate on your own feelings. For instance, "Even though I'm feeling (controlled not appreciated, unloved and unattractive)" is the perfect way to begin. Here's how to pinpoint the issue.

Step 2. Gage your feelings using an index of 1-10.

If you can gauge how intense your emotions are on a scale of one 10 to 1, you allow yourself the opportunity to begin looking at your situation and improvement within the emotions that are dragging you in the current scenario.

It is the best method to make sure you've got an emotion that is strong enough for a successful EFT exercise , but it's the last step to take before you start working on EFT!

Once you have started your journey with EFT You may be tempted by minor issues like anxiety in specific situations.

But, the smaller emotions result from deep-rooted emotions that you've acquired throughout your life.

You'll quickly be able to improve your results if you are patient and have confidence to confront your deeply held emotions instead of slamming out your more pleasant emotions during an hour.

If you'd like to see rapid progress over the course of a few months of effort, be working on EFT each day and act on your emotions using an 8-10 scale for quick change.

However you decide to take on EFT it is certain that you will reap positive results from the sessions you do. If you make sure your energy is high, you'll be able to smash through and repair thousands of emotions that can take several months to unravel.

If you can identify the most fundamental emotion you feel There's a way to increase the intensity of your emotions in the event that the intensity falls below 8. Consider how you could achieve an emotional intensity of 10. If your intensity does not change to an 8then Repeat the exercise twice more...if you're still not experiencing any emotional intensity greater than 8 after the third attempt to raise your intensity, finish the exercise in your final attempt to increase the intensity of your emotions.

Step 3: The open tap!

Once you've pinpointed an emotion that is deeply rooted and you've identified a deep emotion, it's time for tapping! This process is simple and is the first step in tapping. The first tap begins by hitting to the KC (or karate chop). This helps the brain to recognize the experience and emotion you're trying to resolve to focus your attention on what is important to you during the workout.

This is known as the setup!

....

....

The first part of the set-up could be done in two ways:

#1. You can apply an external scenario, such as "Even when my partner attempts to influence me, ..."

#2. It is possible to address your responses to situations like this "Even when I feel I'm not valued by my beloved ,..."

....
....

The second half of the set-up can be carried out in three different ways:

1 "Even even though it is difficult for me to feel (personal reaction) I sincerely and totally admit to myself."

With the help of"feel" or the "feel" by using the active "feel" your own personal reactions.

2 "Even even (external situation) I love my self, and appreciate and support myself."

If you say"even though (insert name, followed by by a specific action) You'll be addressing external friction.

3 "Even regardless of (any situation) I'm not happy, I love me and respect myself.

Simple versions work to any task.

....

....
....

It is essential that your established phrase is in a negative. Although positive thoughts are beneficial and common all through your lifetime, EFT is a little different once you start the process. The first objective of EFT is to address directly the issues that are causing negativity in your life and release the blockages in the flow of energy.

An excellent example of how to phrase it in a negative way is when you are procrastinating: If, for instance, you're putting off your work, do not say "Even even though I've done something three times in the past week," I sincerely acknowledge and cherish myself.. Instead, you should say "Even even though I'm scared of losing my loved ones as I devote my time and energy to the goals I have set, but I completely respect and cherish myself."

This will enable you to deal with the issues that are taking place within your energy system, and will help you identify the root of the issue you're trying to resolve.

*THE OPENING TAPE: TAP The TAP KC (THE KARATE CHOP POINT) and repeat your phrase 3 times.

If you live your life on a day every day, remaining positively and positive is a great way to reach your goals and be satisfied. But, when negative feelings are bound to arise during your journey towards becoming a more joyful and healthy person, you can just write them down and deal with these issues in the morning, during your breaks, or in the evening, before you go to bed. This method lets you break through the limiting beliefs of you and also deal with your feelings towards past hurts that aren't working for your current situation.

The first tap allows you to frame your goal of healing the particular cut during exercise.

While it's vital to be positive and maintain a positive attitude and addressing negative emotions in a direct manner the normal state of flow will take place.

The effectiveness of EFT is in identifying the negative emotions you experience and address them so you can think and behave in a positive manner. The effect of EFT are amazing when used in this manner.

Fourth step: the pattern of tapping.

Taps are the mainstay of an EFT system. This step lets you successfully complete a full cycle of EFT and helps to correct the energy and nervous system on a molecular. Once you know the proper emotion and the appropriate phrase to apply, it's time to start the major part of the EFT procedure.

APRIL 15 - AFTER EVERY CIRCUIT OR SESSION It's important to drink A LASSER OF WATER to stay hydrated.

EFT releases the tightness and restrictions in your body that been previously blocked. The opening to your body's energy flow permits oxygen and water to enter the areas of your body that are famished prior to exercise. Drinking an enormous glass or container of fluid, you enable your body to replenish its own health and prepare for the next exercise.

One session per day is enough to allow you to reap all the advantages EFT can bring to your life, if you decide to do seven sessions at a time you'll enjoy the ease of finishing a circuit.

A great program to deal with an cellular memory that is deeply rooted is according to:

The first step in the plan is to complete 7 consecutive sessions once you've identified the problem you'd like to address. Be sure to drink one glass of water at the session has ended. 7

When you've completed the first circuit, you will be able to continue for the remainder of the week working on a single circuit in the morning , and later at night.

Each week, you should revisit the circuit and allow yourself to fully engage in improving the energy systems of your body.

Repeat the process over 3 months or until you're completely free of the emotion you are experiencing.

Step 5: Examine the intensity level of the previous test.

When you've completed your first circuit, the intensity of the topic you're working on will decrease. In most cases, you'll reach a plateau between 1-4 however these plateaus can be easily overcome if you complete your workout in a disciplined manner.

Although it's advised to lower your intensity to a level of zero but it's essential to keep up with your training on a daily routine.

When people begin to practice EFT you'll see an immediate improvement following a session. It takes time to get rid of the deeply-rooted emotions that are a part of your.

It can take up to three months to completely overpower your most negative emotions , so don't become down if you're feeling stuck after a couple of weeks.

Each week, you should take note of your progress in the general happiness you feel inside of you. If you're lucky, when you've completed a year of EFT practice, you'll experience an unnatural joy and happiness levels of 7 or higher.

Chapter 3: Emotional Overeating

Food, Stress And Emotions

It is not just about eating to satisfy your cravings. Many people seek food to find relief, comfort, or satisfaction. But, this type of eating pattern won't help you overcome your emotional issues. This can only cause you to feel worse afterward. The original problem persist and lingers, but there could also feel guilt over having eaten too often.

Recognizing the triggers of emotional eating could assist you in overcoming the habit of overeating and unhealthy food cravings. In the long term this will also assist you follow your diet plan correctly.

Emotional eating

Emotional eating refers to the use of food in order to make you feel better.

In essence, this means that you eat food so that you can satisfy your emotional needs , not eating food to take in more food. Sometimes, eating food as a way to express joy or as a way to reward, or even as a way to recharge yourself isn't necessarily an issue.

If you turn to food as your primary mental coping strategy then you'll eventually be stuck in a particular type of unhealthy pattern where you will never be able to address the real issue.

It is not easy to satisfy your hunger with food. While you're at it eating, it can make you feel better. But the feelings that led you to have a snack in the first instance remain. Sometimes, you'll be feeling worse than you experienced because you consumed much more than what you needed. Then, you may blame yourself for allowing your desire and not being able to fight it.

This could eventually exacerbate the root of the issue. In the end you'll stop learning more about the best ways to how to handle your feelings. In the end, it can make you feel helpless about your feelings as well as the food you consume.

How do you differentiate the difference between physical hunger and emotional hunger

Before using the technique of emotional freedom to deal with emotional eating first you must know how to distinguish the physical and emotional.

It's more complicated than you think. This is particularly relevant if you are using food as a way to treat your problems regularly.

Since emotional hunger is a powerful force it can be difficult to misinterpret this with your physical hunger.

Luckily, there are indications to seek out:

A sudden feeling of emotional hunger appears. It hits you immediately and can feel overwhelming and urgent. overwhelming.

A feeling of hunger can make people want to eat certain kinds of comfort foods.

The hunger that this type of person experiences can cause you to eat without thinking.

It is difficult to be satisfied until you are satisfied.

The emotion of hunger doesn't come from your stomach.

The desire to feel emotionally full can cause guilt, shame or regret.

Different people consume food because of different motives. The first step to stop the habit of eating out for emotional reasons is to pinpoint your triggers.

If you take this approach it will help you reduce the anxiety you feel as you'll be less inclined to eating whatever you want at random times.

Chapter 4: Begin Tapping

If you're searching for a quick and easy solution to an issue that isn't addressed by other methods it isn't a problem for you. EFT tapping is often portrayed as a fast fix, but it can be a quick fix at times. Sometimes, emotional issues have to be explored , and there are there are a myriad of methods to be used before the final results are visible. If you find that this is more complicated than you first thought and you're looking to start with the basics There are a few strategies that you could try.

Aiding with Symptoms or Pain Relief by using EFT tapping: The basic recipe can be used to assist with the alleviation of pain or symptoms caused by any injury or condition that is diagnosed. Start by placing the symptoms in the setting and the reminder phrases and then tapping through several rounds of the recipe. Check how severe the pain is prior to and after each session. Utilizing an affirmation technique that was mentioned in the previous chapter and continue until you feel a sense of relief.

If you feel relief, use it as often as you want.

Try describing the pain more precisely for greater relief.

This strategy can be used whenever you need to, but it is best utilized as a temporary remedy. While you may be able to bring the pain down to a minimal level at times, you shouldn't anticipate a zero-per-hour every time. We do not expect long-term outcomes from this method even if it happens to occur in the present and later. If symptoms do return it is possible to look into any emotional concerns.

Always consult your doctor for any medical concerns.

Assistance with Problems with Behavior and Performance by using EFT Tapping The same principle applies as physical discomfort. It addresses any unwelcome behavior or limitations of your performance that could be interpreted as an unresolved emotional problem. The goal of tackling the limit, tapping using the EFT tapping recipe will be the same thing as any physical manifestation.

Make sure you affirm yourself, and then use follow the EFT tapping recipe to begin. If you achieve the desired outcome, you don't need to dig any further. This approach can be utilized whenever you want to.

If you can put yourself in the position which causes the problem, and tap as you feel the pain the process will be more efficient. If not, try to imagine your situation and then generate intenseness, then follow the fundamental recipe to lessen the level of intensity. You may notice that the next time you're in the same circumstance, the intensity is significantly lower than the normal.

Like the physical manifestations, do not count on that the intensity will be at zero every time Also, don't expect to see long-term outcomes. If it can help you advance and feel more relaxed, try it whenever you'd like to.

If this method doesn't yield the desired results Then identifying and fixing the emotional factors is your next step. Finding the emotional problems that affect your performance could be as simple as thinking about the circumstances that led to the issue first started. It is possible that you recall the words your loved ones was saying or perhaps you remember feeling snubbed, humiliated or dismissed at some point.

Curing Fears using EFT tapping: Spaces that are enclosed and crowds, flying insects, public speaking and heights are just a few of the common fears that must be addressed. Start by thinking about what you are afraid of and determine the level of your fear. Utilize the recipe that is the foundation to help you feel better.

Put yourself in a real-life situation. In front of a crowd, climb a step ladder or find a spider, and examine if the intensity has changed. If it is still high then tap the screen before proceeding.

If your fear resurfaces examine the root of any emotional causes.

People tend to use the term phobia loosely. If you've been diagnosed with a phobia it's not just an isolated. Consider seeking assistance from a professional.

Curbing your cravings by EFT tapping It doesn't matter whether you are food, potato chips alcohol, cigarettes, sugar chocolate, or any other addictive behavior. Start by following the recipe at any time you feel the urge.

If this helps lessen the cravings, test it out when cravings start to appear. The basic recipe may lessen the cravings. Craving is one of the lesser forms of addiction. If you are addicted to any drug such as alcohol, cigarettes or other behavior is likely to suffer from more severe issues.

Helping Parents, Children, and teachers with EFT tapping Teachers and parents who face occasional behaviors issues or assist children in regaining their focus can utilize the base recipe to address whatever problem you are facing.

You may need to change the affirmation to ensure that it is a representation of the issue from the right perspective, however the majority of children respond to the energy work.

At home, parents can tap their phones during the times when their children tell them about the problems they faced during the day. In helping children process experiences as they occur and not storing the disruptions is an excellent present to children.

If you have a diagnosis of any kind that require treatment, like Autism asperger's, ADD, Dyslexia, or any other ongoing trauma, you'll need to find a professional training. We would like to see that one day every school will have an EFT nurse or counselor who can assist the children.

Treatment of physical diseases through EFT Tapping: Apply the same method to treat symptoms or pain whenever discomfort appears. Any chronic or diagnosed condition involves the treatment of emotional triggers. There could be physical reasons which EFT will not help. One theory is that carrying the burden of many years of stress or problems can make our bodies more susceptible to illness, and we have to eliminate all the stress we can.

Assistance for PTSD as well as War Veterans with EFT Tapping: PTSD or Post Traumatic Stress Disorder are the result of one or more traumatizing events. In many instances, we can find a solution to the cause of the disturbance by aiming at the fundamentals of the incident. For Veterans certain events seem obvious, yet they can be extremely painful. If you're experiencing difficult memories, but think you are able to work through them all without creating more discomfort, take it slow and focus on one at one moment.

Whatever you decide to do, make sure you use EFT with the help of a qualified professional to make sure you are receiving the correct help.

We recognize the need to aid Veterans after they return from the war, however PTSD is not something an average person or your neighbor can try to solve. You should take your Vet and their family members to specialists if required.

Certain PTSD cases could have a long-standing time of minor traumas. These can be difficult to manage. If you require assistance to make sense of your past There are many professionals trained to do this.

Treating emotional problems by using EFT Tapping: Nearly people today have a problem to tackle that's built on an emotional base. Self-esteem issues, social anxiety work stress, relationship problems or anger management can be just a few examples. These terms may appear to be specific, but they are EFT phrases. The most efficient method of getting results is by following the basic recipe and then addressing the feelings related to the issue.

If you're having issues with your relationship Think about what your partner has done to cause you the anger and let it go.

When you are dealing with anger management issues take a look at it was that led you to be angry, and then take that anger out.

Social anxiety, stress at work or anything else that triggers emotional stress can be tackled using the same basic formula. You can tackle these issues whenever they arise the same way as you would unwelcome behavior or physical signs.

Finding Peace in Yourself Finding Peace in Your Life with EFT tapping. The principal aim is the freedom of your emotions. Everyone wants immediate relief from the aches of our lives, however for anything rapid fixes, they're not an end-to-end solution. The promotion of peace through solving issues of the past and tackling all new issues without causing any more interruptions is the aim. No matter what type of issue you're experiencing You might want to consider making use of EFT to help you stay on track with a treatment to improve your emotional well-being. You should learn to utilize EFT methods frequently.

Common common sense No matter what you've read about EFT and its ability to help you solve issues fast. The actual results will be quicker and more efficient for cases that are simple. If you've already been diagnosed as having a mental or medical issue, your situation could not be a straightforward one. The process of improvement can be achieved by seeking out long-term help from a professional. EFT could yield some results even when there is no other method to aid. The expectation of a quick solution to chronic or diagnosed illness. is not a reasonable expectation.

Beware: If you are aware about a long-standing history of trauma that has led to your symptoms, are recognized as suffering from a health issue or your pain is ongoing and persistent, the EFT procedure will be more complex. It could cause you to be more uncomfortable before you begin to improve. The reason behind this is EFT is more effective than you think. Learn all you can and work on your emotional problems. If you're not getting the results you'd like or if the tapping is beginning to cause you stress consider seeking help by an expert.

You've learned a few helpful techniques to get started with the fundamentals of EFT.

The recipe's basic formula could be applied to many different but common problems.

Start by directing the tapping on the problem to test if it works. If not, study more and go further.

If you've had a diagnosis or history of trauma or a history of trauma, the process is more complex. These tips might not provide lasting relief. You may require more advanced techniques of EFT.

A certified EFT practitioner can help you in your healing, regardless of the issue you're facing.

Chapter 5: Methods For Finding

Tapping Points

The first step of the use of EFT is to understand the tapping points, also known as meridians. The free ebook included in this book illustrates these points for you to study. Additionally, there are a variety of online resources and videos to identify these points. Be sure to tap with a firm force however, not too hard to cause injury! Alongside the tapping, you'll also have to affirm yourself. In future chapters and will include suggested phrases to apply.

Tapping should be done in specific areas for the most effective healing process and to free yourself from emotional burdens. It is recommended to tap four to five times on each spot and then affirm it with a positive mantra (to be explained in chapter 5) to reap the maximum benefits. Furthermore, tapping needs to be done in the right order to achieve optimal outcomes. Here are the tapping points , and are in the sequence in which they should be used.

The first point to tap is on the highest point of the skull. The tap is performed by placing fingers in a reversed position over the top of the skull. The tapping of this point can stimulate the energy system since numerous meridians cross at this point . It is also the area that you will find the 7th Chakra is found that is the point of entry for all the energy flowing to our body. Tapping this point can help you let go of your inner critic and lack of concentration. Additionally, this posture assists in increasing clarity as well as intuition, focus in addition to spiritual connection. The acupressure Meridian also known as the "Hundred Meeting Points'" Meridian.

The second place is in the middle of your eyebrows, which is just over and to the left from the nostril. The tapping of this spot can bring peace and spiritual healing , as it relieves tension, sadness and anger. The acupressure Meridian also known as the Bladder Meridian.

The third position of tapping is located on the bone that runs along the outer corner of the eyes. It can be found on the outer edge of the brow, since it's the boney protrusion that reaches the temple's edge. This is the position that releases the fear of change, anger and resentment, it allows compassion and clarity to flow through. It's often referred to as the 'Gall Bladder Meridian.

To determine the fourth place you need to tap the bone beneath the eye, just 1 millimetre below the pupils. This tap will aid in the release of anxiety or anxiety, sadness, and anxiety. But, tapping this area can also help in bringing feeling of safety and calm to move forward. This is known in the "Stomach' Meridian.

The fifth tap position is situated directly below the nose, inside the tiny indentation close to the top of your lip. This is a position that eliminates feelings of shame, guilt and grief, as well as fears of failure, fear , or embarrassment, as well as psychological reverses. It also aids feelings of self-acceptance and compassion and self-confidence. This is also known as the 'Governing' Meridian.)

The chin is where you will find the site for the 6th tapping spot. It is situated under the lip, and is in the dimple between the lip's bottom as well as the chin. The chin point will assist in letting go of doubt, being unsure of yourself or being confused. It will assist in allowing for confidence in your certainty, clarity, and self-acceptance. This is known as the Central meridian.

The seventh tap point is called the Collar Bone Point. It's located right below the collarbone's knob and just behind the indentation that lies below the Adam's apple. This point is recommended to alleviate stress, indecision anxiety, worries, the feeling of being stuck, and psychological reverses. It also gives certainty, clarity and the ability to make a move with ease. It is often referred to as the "Kidney Meridian"..

Eighth tapping is also known in the field of the Under Arm Point. You can locate this point by placing your finger for at minimum six inches beneath the armpit. Women may find it easier by following the straps of their bra. Fear, guilt, doubt as well as low self-esteem and despair can be released through tapping this area. Therefore, calmness as well as confidence and clarity are also possible. The meridian that is in play is known as the "Spleen Meridian"..

Tapping on the "Inner Gate" can help relieve nausea, anxiety and nerves, as well as carpal tunnel discomfort. This is in the inner part and outside of each wrist. It can be found by taking the measurement of the width of three fingers upwards from the wrist's crease. This is the point that connects to one of the yin channels in the upper part that connect the heart, pericardium and the lungs.

Another essential tapping technique to master is the "karate chop". It can be found on the soft, fleshy portion of your hand that isn't dominant connecting the finger's base as well as your wrist. This position is commonly employed in the EFT setup, basic tapping techniques, and for psychological reverses. The tapping position assists in psychological reversals that result from feeling stuck, refusing to change, and having the inability to let go, and intense feelings of sorrow, sadness, fear, vulnerability and compulsive behaviour. It assists in healing from loss, getting rid of things as well as people who do not serve your highest interests and aids in bringing you into current moment. It is also known as the "Small Intestine Meridian.

Chapter 6: Achieving Peace For Everyone-Advanced Eft

After you've mastered the basics of EFT method, and have practiced the technique until it is perfect then it's time to progress to the more advanced EFT technique, which is known as ad Personal Peace Process (PPP). It is the core healing process of each person. Spiritual counselors, therapists doctor, or other physical or emotional healing individual can also utilize this technique, since it has been proven to be an effective instrument.

The process

PPP involves creating a list of all things that cause you stress in your life and then slowing tap these events, and then removing the negative events from our lives. If done with diligence, we can remove the negativity that is a part of our life and eliminate all the causes of physical and emotional ailments. The result is personal peace. This helps to accelerate your progress towards making peace in the world.

The benefits of PPP

* Speeds up healing and enhances the efficacy when used as an addition to sessions conducted by an therapist or physician

When it is done regularly it can assist in getting rid of the emotional baggage you've collected over time. A more positive self-image and a greater sense of liberation with less self-doubt are possible by doing this

PPP is a powerful method to prevent serious disease instances that can occur in people. The anxiety, fear and anger that dwell in you over time could manifest into disease. If EFT tapping targets these issues and you are able to prevent these illnesses.

* It can be employed as a way of determining the root of the issue. If you can eliminate negative aspects in yourself then you would have included the most important issues in a way.

* It's excellent to have a consistent and efficient way of relaxing and can serve to set an example for others to follow.

PPP defined

The majority of the physical and emotional issues we face are the result of situations that haven't been properly resolved. These situations can be effectively dealt with by using EFT. When used correctly by the practitioner and the patient it can improve healing rates quickly and decreases the cost associated with treatment.

While medicines do play an important role in the treatment of diseases but when the root cause for the disease is treated by EFT The resolution becomes higher and the speed is also faster.

EFT is able to eliminate all negativity that is residing in our minds which results in a greater chance of success. Although it's been proven beneficial for ailments like trauma, headaches, and phobias, it could be utilized for general conditions like depression, anxiety as well as low self-esteem and the chronic insomnia and feelings of being unloved.

If you can eliminate all emotional conflicts that reside in your head then you will have fewer internal conflicts to confront. This leads to personal peace. The process of personal peace is distinct in that it tackles problems in which traditional healing techniques have not been able to resolve.

The physical impact PPP

The personal peace process is not only a powerful method of emotional healing also addresses physical illnesses too. Disorders like digestive problems, Cancer, breathing problems headaches, AIDS and so on. are treated effectively. It is well-known that the physical problems are caused by not resolved traumas, anger, guilt, grief and other feelingshas been proven in a scientific manner. This is why the many treatments and drugs employed in conventional treatment have not worked. The medications are only used to disguise the effects. However, EFT and its other techniques are proving to be effective in healing and are used as complement methods to treat the root cause of disease effectively.

The process

1. Make a list of every event that has troubled you. If you don't have at least 50 points or more, that means you're not doing it with a sense of humour and that is why people typically find hundreds of similar problems.

2. Certain events might not be causing any pain to you right now. However, you should note them down. If you can still recall the details, it indicates that they require resolution.

3. Give a name to each item or event on the list, such as

* My brother struck me in the yard.

* I stole Clara's pencil

* I nearly fell in the front of the truck when driving recklessly

* The entire school laughed over my ridiculous speech

* Mom was not willing to speak to me for a week

4. Once you've finished the list, pick the most important issues from the list and use EFT for each one until you are no longer contemplating them, or, at the very least, can be amused by them. Keep applying EFT to an incident until the issue is removed. If you're unable to reach the 0-10 degree of intensity for any issue, you must use at least 10 EFT sessions that address the issue from every angle that you can imagine. When the most pressing problems have been resolved then you can move onto the next most important issue on the list.

5. You must deal with at least one to three issues each day. If you continue to do this over three months, you will

have resolved more than 250 problems. Then you'll begin to notice the improvements that the resolution created. You won't get frustrated, angry or stressed quickly. Your body will feel more comfortable and more hydrated. The majority of issues you faced would have gone away completely. Physical issues like pulse, breathing, and blood pressure are normalized.

6. The mental and physical health you'll feel could lead you to consider quitting all medications you're taking. However, don't stop taking medications unless your doctor recommends it.

This Personal Peace Procedure If used properly it can offer you an numerous relief options. This easy and efficient method is a powerful tool, and makes it an effective instrument for people who have deeply rooted and unresolved issues.

Chapter 7: The Set-Up Phrase

The EFT Set-Up mantra was created to signal your body and subconscious to know that tapping had begun. It also assists your conscious mind concentrate on the goal. It also helps you focus your mind. Karate Chop point has been considered to "wake" your body and make it ready for new information and stimuli.

From the humble beginnings of tapping a couple of decades ago, a guiding principle came into existence that was designed to help. Keep in mind that the Set-Up concept was first introduced at the beginning of tapping, and like many other things in life and belief systems, grew into more dogmatic. It's not a reason to disqualify its value. In fact, we're exploring the possibility of traps which can get you caught in the EFT tracks.

I have personally put down the Set-Up Phrase a while ago. The one you've heard of that is an abbreviation of something similar to this:

"Even although I'm suffering from (this issue)

I am still deeply and totally

Accept and love myself regardless."

This could lead to psychological reverse

It's true I did it. It could be difficult due to the fact that you might not:

Absolutely and deeply love yourself.

Completely or deeply love yourself.

Accept yourself completely and fully.

Accept yourself completely or deeply.

Completely and deeply forgive yourself.

Take a deep breath OR completely forgiving yourself.

You may be experiencing feelings of self-loathing or not being accepted, of anger, or fear or pain over doing something or being afraid to do in the most dire situations.

When your mind detects how intense and totally you feel, you imagine it makes a slight chuckle or tells you: "

H

"Yeah, right" and then turns around to look at you with"Yeah, Right" and then says "Good luck with

that

If you're one of the people who - at this moment and right now - isn't completely and totally

with

Yourself, the typical setup phrase could stop genuine healing from happening.

If you remember, I mentioned previously that not all Reversals are internal. This is an example of a genuine, heartfelt effort to help EFT experts and philosophers assist but it comes with consequences that could be detrimental to.

How can you determine what setup you have in mind will be a good fit for your needs? Easy. Do a truthful statement and observe how you feel. All you need is total honest, sometimes brutal, truth. Make use of to use the SUDs (Subjective units of distress) measurement. On a scale from 10 to 0 how true do these statements seem to you?

I am awestruck by myself.

I absolutely love myself.

I am incredibly happy with myself.

I am completely comfortable with myself completely.

I am deeply sorry for myself.

I have completely forgiven myself completely.

Let

Let's take as an example to show what could happen with an imaginary character.

I am awestruck by myself. AUD levels of 8. "I find myself to be pretty good. I would like to be slightly more or less ..."

I absolutely love myself. Seven SUDs. "I would not say that I am"I'm 100. I've made a few mistakes that I am really sorry for and haven't completely forgiven myself for the things I've done."

I deeply respect myself. Six SUDs. "I know many people who claim they have however I am not convinced of it. That's how I feel but not completely open to."

I fully accept myself completely. Four SUDs. "No one is really able to fully accept their own. Except sociopaths. Yes, I'm not.

T

I completely accept myself. I was at a point where I could completely accept myself. ..."

I am deeply sorry for myself. Five SUDs. "

I

I've accepted my own forgiveness for a number of things, but there's always more to be done."

I am completely sorry for myself completely. I am completely forgiven. "

Nope. It's not true.

The things I did that nobody forced me to do that burden my conscience. It was that time ... The person ... Ah and I said ..."

In my case, I deliberately did not make this an extreme case since the majority of us's inner lives aren't particularly extreme.

76

It's not worth the risk to overstate. In fact, it could cause things to be a million billion trillion times more expensive.

What happens when you are infatuated with exaggeration?

"Tapping isn't working for me."

"Tapping was no longer working."

"EFT doesn't work."

I'm experiencing an EFT Failure."

What we learn from this fundamental understanding is that you can't learn the setup phrase over and over and then repeating it repeatedly without thinking could cause it's own issues.

In the above example, the six sentences all have a level of trouble and must be identified and tackled. In reality, I've employed the set-up formula to aid those who have been stuck and are unable to draw no conclusions about what the issue might be. On the surface it's very helpful since the SUDs reveal the true situation inside the body. Test it out, and discover how it can benefit you.

Sometimes, a surprising benefit is a result of an unintentional issue.

Once we've identified the issues, which may take a while, since we've all been able to create or respond to these issues, I may (but very rarely) utilize an alternative version if I believe it will assist.

"For me to truly love myself, I'd have to ..."

The results can be instructive even though they appear as negative. They could look at the problems from a different perspective and could reveal new avenues to follow.

Are you one of those who have 'never recovered from it' and basically live the experience every day? They have nothing progress. There's no way to get there.

Right now

There's no way out from the 'then'. For the majority of us, fortunately the way is much more straightforward.

Before we are able to completely and totally let go, it is necessary to understand the things we're willing to let go of. Finding those answers may take some time and effort, but neither are reasons not to attempt.

We humans are known for searching to find meaning in everything, it may take time to establish an entirely new perspective. A lot of people, including myself cannot or won't be satisfied with just knowing about the issue. They should be aware of the reason why there is was an issue. Sometimes, it's impossible to truly are aware of the reason.

If you were faced with a decision to make, you could identify the issue and resolve it, or identify the issue and then prolong it by searching for a meaning which is likely remain elusive for a a longer period, what option would you pick?

I would get myself in knots trying to find the deeper meaning behind some issues. Certain of them were particularly frustrating because , despite my best efforts try, nothing came up. Nothing. Not even a whisper. It occurred to me that I had gotten myself free from the initial issue and was building a new. Again I attempted modification, and it did the trick.

"Even although I've experienced this issue I'm not sure the reason why it happened and it's causing me anxiety, so I'm ready to let go of that uncomfortable sensation." Sometimes, a small tendril would appear and I'd realize that it was tangibly connected to the issue I had was able to solve, so I'd gently tap it out. Other times, I let go of the idea that there are things that aren't known.

EFT solves problems. Why should we create a new?

Every now and then we need a reminder that we could be the creators of our own suffering.

This Buddhist poem is a popular reminder of the burden we bear on our own, and the ways we can shift the burden to bear it on other people.

A monk who was old and a younger one were walking through the forest when they saw an elderly woman who was standing near an eddy, crying as she was scared to traverse the river. Without saying anything, the monk who was old grabbed her and carried her to the other side the stream, placing her on the other side. He then continued walking without saying a word. After an hour, the young monk remarked: "I can't believe you touched her!" Without missing a step, the old monk responded with a smile: "I can't believe you're still carrying her."

The koan is a way to bring the reader to the next thought which is that time has taught me that we can make the seemingly simple seem complicated. We can explode our own transgressions to such a degree that they have any resemblance to the reality. It is also possible to similarly do it even if we're the one who committed the offense. This is not a way to make any light of the important issues that individuals have endured or committed.

Most of us, all times we can improve the situation by preventing it from getting worse.

There's a method used in the work of Steve Wells in Australia that employs gentle humor to address certain issues by making the story absurd and, in turn, giving the perspective of a different person. I suggest you check out his work. I've provided a URL to his website at the at the end of this book.

The question of perspective is vital. I think that for the majority of people it's important to be aware of when you should not tap. Marathons can be a great experience for somepeople, however for others, they're not just physically exhausting, but can also cause over-identification or exaggeration of the issue.

I'm guessing that the setup phrase is an optimistic exaggeration or a play on "fake it until you can get it'

. I

I'll talk about tapping scripts and their problems during the forthcoming chapter.

At times, when I helped people tap ideas, I realized that regardless of how simple I made it, there were some who were so used to scripts that they would email me asking for me to repeat the words I had stated. It's possible to unlock the cage, but that doesn't mean that the lion will leave the cage and go out to freedom.

With that said, since the"set-up" phrase could be unproductive, I'm required to suggest a method of alternative, but I'd like to make it clear that I don't believe this as a script, and neither should you.

Instead of starting with a rote statement begin by taking an in-depth sounding. You can either pinpoint what you need to focus on or, if nothing else comes to mind, you can discern your current emotions.

I'm feeling confused and don't know what's going on."

Begin tapping. There is no need to make use of a dialogue running. You're aware of your feelings so tap. If you aren't able to identify an emotional issue, but you're experiencing a general feeling of being 'off', it could be because there's no emotional reason that is causing it. Take a look at this:

"Even even though I'm feeling slightly lost and don't know why, but I'm willing to let pass." Then you'll experience an insight flash. "

I'm feeling lost because I'm exhausted. I'm tired because I did not sleep well. I couldn't get a good night's sleep due to the fact that I ate a lot of cheese."

I'm not trying to minimize any issue that makes someone feel bad however, sometimes we think that we are more involved than the issue really has. This is why I'm an advocate of internal honesty and a detachment from over-exaggeration.

I've witnessed and met individuals who, when asked to define the SUDs they experience on an issue, will unquestionably refer to it as "

11

" on the scale of 10. It's not helpful. I can understand why it hurts, it's overwhelming, and that it's an enormous issue that's impacted an arterial, but it's not an 11.

Most likely, people will be able to tolerate it for a short time because they sympathize with your pain, but use too much of it, and it can bring your credibility to the forefront. Are you trying to win your sympathy? Do you want to trick me into feeling more pity for you than I do? Do you want to be noticed? Are you controlling?

In the example of cheese, the sensation was traced back to an environmental cause which is why you shouldn't rule them out. There are a variety of triggers from the environment, in addition to new, undiagnosed or recognized health problems. If you're a person with spiritual beliefs, even certain ideas available could cause discomfort. We'll look at a few in the future.

Utilize EFT according to the way it is most effective for you.

I've witnessed too many people getting caught by the terms that should be used, correct timing of tapping, as well as other "rules" that aren't even rules even. Gary Craig, who brought EFT to the world and has always believed that tapping is a process that is constantly evolving and experimental. I'm with Gary Craig. A new idea does not indicate that an evolution step has taken place. It's not an unidirectional way from 'there' to'

.

As I started looking back in the mists of 1998 , there was only a tiny amount of information in comparison to the current volume. The data I gathered was a bit experimental and there was a sense of the rules that were being developed were more of an unexpected: "Well, that worked and appears to be going at it."

I'm urging you to go to that state, is for you. EFT is beginning to emerge

You've tried several things that worked, some that didn'twork, and a few which were confusing. Take a fresh start and fill it in with the items you're sure worked for you before you first started. Then, hopefully inspired by this, you can build the foundation of the potential of

P

Oral

Freedom the way you want it

echnique.

Instead of a set-up word, the procedure I have used and have utilized with other users is straightforward since it is what it has to be.

The first step is to determine If you are able to identify the issue.

If not, begin with your feelings.

If you are feeling mixed emotions Start with the most intense one.

If you aren't able to decide which is your strongest option, begin wherever you want to.

Start tapping.

Begin with any aspect. You could adhere to this EFT recipe or simply go to the specific point or points that resonate with you.

If you're unable to physically tap the points, place your hands over your stomach or the heart, or imagine tapping the points. (I've witnessed this process in a hospital setting where individuals that wanted tapping physically incapable or immobile. I've also used EFT on someone who was suffering from seizures in the airport, and it made me think about the issue of consciousness and mobility with EFT.)

Make it easy. Even even if you just simply say "This sensation" ..." is a good feeling" and then tap on a point

You're listening and doing something valuable.

It's essential to be open to letting things go. Certain people are enslaved to their pain, or aren't sure who they would have been without the pain. Therefore, they seek relief, but not total freedom. A kind treatment for emotional pain, rather than total freedom.

Choose what you would like for yourself and be open about the goal. The management of emotional pain is a lot simpler to access because it is more accessible to the public.

Let

Let's see if we can connect it all with an illustration.

UDS of six.

Tapping the collarbone.

"This feeling. It's a feeling that I'm not able to describe.

You can't find.

In the face.

"I feel worried. I'm worried that the plan don't go according to plan."

Chin.

(Nothing is more that than that.)

The arm is under the table.

"This feeling. What ever it's about, I'm ready for it to go."

Under the eyes.

I'm glad I can let this go."

The top part of head.

(Nothing else than that.)
Karate chop.

"It's secure to release it."

SUDs check for 4, which means it's working even though we don't understand what it's doing. You'll notice that we're using these points in a way that is intuitive rather than rote and I intentionally confused them. If you're confused, try following the Basic Recipe or come up with Your own basic recipe.

The key ingredients are:

Tap wherever you feel led to tap. You are your body. Your brain and your emotions, your personal rules. I've witnessed several (too numerous) people get lost and overwhelmed when they don't remember the exact points to tap in which order. Relax the pressure and decide which taps to use.

If you are able to, describe the sensation to whatever extent you are able, regardless of how tiny.

I think that the thing that is the force behind EFT is

Willingness

to let things let things go. The thought drew you in the beginning because it seemed to you that there was something lacking or there was just excessive of something you wanted to get rid of. I'd like to make it clear that we shouldn't confuse intentions (a prospective plan or a hopeful goal) with the concept of the concept of willingness (the determination to do something about something or fulfill a need). Let's make it a point to be willing. The plan can be formulated later, after we've cleaned up some space.

Are you able to do that? Are you able to just be willing?

This is the best way I can provide you with and I hope that you'll take it.

The words don't matter. They can't save you from yourself particularly if they're somebody who's words and you're trying make yourself fit into a mold which wasn't designed to fit you.

Select a few keywords or simple phrases to aid you. Try to recall other people's information can cause you to lose focus on your own. There is an internal conversation. We all do. Make use of it, and do it as you would normally. Every word is in play. If you like dropping the occasional F-bomb in your day-to-day life, you can make sure to add some more in your EFT practice. I'm not sure what Higher Power you believe in will pour gasoline on you and light a match to the use of swear words during EFT. It's your Higher Power that has all day accomplish this.

I

I've discovered that "let let it go" is extremely effective for me and those I've assisted with, so please try it with your unique flavors to it. Try "release secure, safe it's time to let go to let it go let it go, but I'm not able to'" and add "let let it go". My own results started to rise as I began to do this. Later, I discovered an American man America, Robert Smith, who came up with FasterEFT and employs the same principles and certain terms and phrases. I'm not familiar with his method, but it could be worth looking into.

Reminder

S

:

EFT gives you the best chance possible to attain inner peace in your daily life. It's always personal and all about YOU. Your task is to try out and adapt the EFT methods to align with the most effective routes and the least resistance to you.

If "tapping isn't working for me"

I

It will change until it is.

If "tapping does not work" I could also look for new ways of using it to my advantage.

If "EFT doesn't work"

It

This is because I'm using a design that was designed to be a fit for the needs of someone else.

Chapter 8: Applying Eft Tapping To Address Specific Issues

One of the most frequent issues that arise when you start tapping to reduce your cravings for food to lose weight is if you recall the place, image or person who your cravings bring back. When you tap it is essential be extra careful in taking note of any negative thoughts that pop up. Pay attention, too, to any thoughts that come that come from your subconscious.

These thoughts can hinder your ability to take the next step in EFT and stop you from achieving your goals. If you're not able to deal with these issues on a personal basis and effectively, you won't succeed in achieving your goal of losing weight or becoming the inner peace or whatever you would like to conquer.

The answer is simple. While using EFT it is important to accept whatever your self-critical thoughts might be and then you must embrace and love yourself while tapping your meridians.

The problem isn't just the food cravings but rather the affection and attention that you require from someone like your mother or dad. When you didn't get. It caused you to be sad or angry. Then you resorted to eating cakes or whatever you can find to make up for the attention you did not receive. This could be described as eating out for emotional reasons.

The subconscious is full of power, but it is possible to use EFT to transform negative feelings and thoughts it tries to instill into your mind's conscious by substituting them with positive thoughts and emotions.

How to tap your way to achieving your Aims

The inquiry process can be an effective tool for identifying the hidden obstacles that keep you from achieving the outcomes you desire. This is a powerful method to uncover the emotions, thoughts and images that could hinder you from doing what you would like to accomplish.

Keep in mind that your conscious brain sets your goals, but it's from your subconscious mind that ideas and thoughts start. Therefore, if you have goals that you would like to accomplish, however, no matter what your efforts, don't attain them There could be an issue with your subconscious. It is possible that you are not using the power of your subconscious.

Uncovering Unconscious Blocks

For instance, if are trying to shed weight, write down the weight you wish to shed. You must ensure that you're particular and clear about your objectives. This is the goal in mind.

Once you have set your intention in your mind and written the goals negative thoughts and feelings may begin to creep in. They can hinder you from achieving your goals. It is possible to think of phrases such as, "Achieving my weight loss goal isn't easy and I'm still a lengthy route to travel" or "It requires an enormous amount of effort but I'm not sure how to go about it" This could begin to control your thoughts.

You can rate the negative thoughts on a scale of 1 to 10 10, with 10, being most powerful or real. It will be a good idea to revisit that score after finishing with a series of tapping sequences. The objective is to lower the score.

Release those unconscious blocks

In the first section, the body contains energy points or meridian points which can be stimulated. You can tap these points to release the negative emotions and feelings. If you are those who are new to tapping, make a tapping pattern like this:

The other hand: "Even though I have many things to accomplish I'm exhausted, and overwhelmed I am grateful and love me." (Repeat the above phrase at least three times.)

Eyes: "I have too much to accomplish."

Eyes outward: "I just cannot do all the things at once."

Under the eye: "It will be a long climb to the top of a hill to shed the pounds."

The upper lip says: "It's a lot of work."

Chin: "I am too overwhelmed and can't find time in my busy schedule time to take on other projects."

Colar bone "You are not able to force me into doing anything else."

The body's side: "I am just too overwhelmed."

The top of the head "This will be tough and I'm certain I won't be able to do it."

Repeat the above process until you can feel the things start to change. Then, try these variations:

Eyes "What If it's not really that difficult?"

Eyes: "What if it will be simple?"

Under the eye: "What if you find it enjoyable."

Lower lip "What do you think if your in awe?"

Chin: "What if it could be stimulating?"

The collar bone "What do you think if you lose weight isn't about working for it, but rather let it go?"

The body's side: "What if you only require to experience and accept your sensations?"

Head of the hair "I embrace and love myself, and everything I feel at the moment."

The goal is uncovering the hidden blocks that prevent you from reaching your objectives. This process will give you the motivation you require, instead of overwhelming you and creating stress. It is about releasing the emotions that are buried in your mind. You can open yourself to more positive and positive possibilities.

Tap to Your Path to Joyful Life

Who doesn't want happiness in their life? It's a known fact that life isn't just a fairytale but you can still feel content even if do not own a flashy sports car or the midst of a massive mansion. Psychotherapists suggest that people need to find happiness with the simplest things. A fulfilling and satisfying life can't be achieved simply by possessing a wealth of possessions or having a successful career on its own.

You could be the most wealthy person on the planet and you'll still be unhappy. As you get to the final chapter in this text, you come realizing that all originates in your subconscious. Emotional feelings are fleeting. Following an initial electric stimulation the nerve impulses start to diminish. They aren't always the source of happiness. If you can find a lasting reason to be happy, you can claim that you've lived a happy life.

Your emotions determine the context

It is now clear that your brain is filled with memories from your various experiences. Every single moment there is an emotion that engulfs your thoughts. It's impossible to control what happens to your life, but you can influence the way you respond to them by instructing your subconscious to transform these negative feelings into positive. The key to feeling good is keeping away from negative feelings.

EFT Tapping Can Help

Negative emotions can make you feel more resentful and anxiety . EFT can help to eliminate those negative thoughts. Be aware that every person is susceptible to the habitual pattern that are based on negative thinking. Once the emotional turmoil inside your own mind is gone then you can begin to be able to feel the peace that is real.

When you begin to alter your mental outlook as you change your perspective, you begin to see issues as issues, challenges, and issues as not threatening to your inner peace. They are simply incidental possibilities.

The freedom from negative thoughts brings You Joy

When you are free of negative feelings and emotions that are preventing the way to inner peace and happiness and inner peace, you will feel an unrestricted joy and joy. Remember that a brand-new sports car is only going to bring you a sense of happiness for a brief period. The joy you experience after you've bought your dream home is only temporary. Positive feelings associated with material possessions don't last, but the feeling of satisfaction you feel inside is a constant feeling. Living a mindful life is the key to a content and happy life.

Mindfulness is all you require to truly take in the joys of life. Yes, it's right to want to possess material goods as these are your benefits for working hard however, your happiness shouldn't be linked to fame and fortune. It should be derived from within.

How to Be Happy? Way to Be Happy

It is not possible for everyone to own an extravagant mansion or automobile. Don't dwell on common notions of a satisfying life. EFT Tapping can save your from worrying about achieving impossible goals. You are special in your own way with gifts and talents that can be utilized to accomplish the goals you would like to accomplish. You might not have the same chance that the man at the White House has but you are able to be successful in your own unique way. You are able to be content wherever you are. Happiness is an attitude!

Chapter 9: What Exactly Is Eft?

Emotional Freedom Technique (EFT) draws from a variety of alternative medicine and acupuncture/acupressure practices, energy medicine, NLP (neuro-linguistic programming) and, a forerunner of EFT, Thought Field Therapy. A person can practice EFT on their own, with therapeutic support , or in an educational workshop.

When participating in the course of an EFT session, a person is able to think deeply about an issue , and taps one bodies "energy meridians" first identified and traced by the ancient Chinese healers and Acupuncturists. EFT practitioners say that a practitioner can make use of these meridians in order to treat and treat a range of physical or psychological ailments by tapping into deep emotional levels. In this way, EFT helps to improve the interaction with the body, mind and energy pathways. There are many proponents who say that when conventional psychological and medical techniques do not work, EFT can work.

What EFT differs from Acupuncture:

Western medicine is focused on the body's complex chemistry and genetic networks, rather than the energy system.

Although EFT utilizes the meridian system of acupuncture however, it doesn't use needles for acupuncture. Chinese medicine recognized the existence of meridians that carry energy 5500 years ago, as per to Steven K. H. Aung and William Pai-Dei Chen ("Clinical Introduction to Medical Acupuncture"). The meridians function as sophisticated electronic circuits in the body. The meridians' circuitry system, similar to that of the nervous system relays information regarding the health of the body.

Acupuncture utilizes more than 300 meridians in the body. It connects energy pathways to organ systems of the body that include kidney liver, spleen or stomach. The meridians used in Chinese Acupuncture also correspond to emotions, like fear, anger, or sadness. While EFT claims that the wisdom of the ancient Chinese wisdom is true, EFT uses only a part of the meridians in order to produce outcomes. That's why EFT is much simpler to master than Acupuncture.

EFT "Basic Recipe":

" At the beginning of the EFT treatment, the person will focus on the things that are most important to him. He might think about psychological physical, physical or performance issues and address them in his mind. Then, he applies his fingers to apply tape to the energy meridians involved for stimulation. A lot of EFT users report significantly quicker results, particularly in comparison to conventional treatment methods. Since no special equipment or tools are required once the person has learned tapping techniques, they can utilize EFT anytime and at anywhere. The basic two-step process to use EFT is known as "The The Basic Recipe."

The human energy bodyis:

Scientists have discovered that our body absorbs into, processes and releases energy. It's electric! The body's energy field is discernable by medical equipment, such as EEG (electroencephalograph) and electrocardiograph (EKG) machines, and by almost every human on a subconscious level. It is not possible for people to "see" the energy of another, however, they certainly feel the energy of a person or individuals each day.

Rupert Sheldrake ("Seven Experiments That can change the world") suggests a few simple tests that anyone can carry out in this area. For instance, when you go on the road, take a look at the vehicle of a driver. This driver always "senses" the interaction and then turns toward the observer. Static electricity is another instance of the body's energetic field in interaction with the surrounding. In a dark area it's sometimes possible to observe electricity leaping from a toe or fingertip. Naturally the nervous system of the body communicates information from the attachments towards the brain. The sensation of pain is an excellent illustration of the flow of electricity throughout the nerve system. It is almost instantaneous due to the energy traveling in the direction of light and electricity.

The study of traditional medicine's energy medicine:

In recent years, a lot of knowledgeable people have investigated alternative therapies are available, like energy medicine and acupuncture. In the end, prominent elite researchers from Harvard, Yale, Columbia and Stanford have been exploring alternative therapies and healing methods.

Research and scientists in the traditional sense aren't completely embracing therapies such as EFT. Yet, research released in The "Journal of Clinical Psychology" (a peer-reviewed journal) and a repeated study by Drs. Harvey Baker and Linda Siegel at Queens College, New York found that EFT's effectiveness was confirmed. The study of 2003 was conducted of S. Wells, P. Polglase, H.B. Andrews, P. Carrington, H.A. Baker ("Evaluation of an intervention that is based on the meridian system EFT/emotional Freedom Techniques") Four out of five evaluations (relating to the relief of anxiety, through breath-controlled deep breathing, and EFT) proved that (via the subjective feedback and lower rate of pulse) EFT outperformed traditional therapies.

David Feistein, Ph.D. ("2012: Review of General Psychology, 'Acupoint stimulation in treating psychological disorders Evidence of efficacy,' 16-368-380. doi

10.1037/a0028602)reports that the "stimulation of acupuncture points (by tapping on, holding, or massaging them) with the activation of a targeted psychological issue...attains positive clinical outcomes in 51 peer-reviewed papers that report on or investigate clinical outcomes following the tapping of acupuncture points to address psychological issues."

Chapter 10: What Is The Cause Of Stress?

Stress is an integral part of every person's life regardless of the place you reside or how much money you earn, or what your social standing. Life can be an adventure, which means that the path that we take isn't always smooth. A bit of stress can help to keep us motivated, and helps us respond to the problems we need to resolve However, too much stress can be dangerous, literally in actual.

Here are a few things that create stress can be found in everyday life:

1.) The school or work setting (meeting requirements, meeting deadlines and other deadlines, etc.)

2.) Relationships (platonic or romantic, family or professional)

3.) Money

4.) Not getting enough rest

5.) Problems with mental or emotional health

6.) Feelings of dreams, passions and goals being achieved

7.) Personal opinions about body image

8.) Not eating , or eating too often

9.) Questions about personal beliefs or beliefs

10.) Making time for everything that needs to be accomplished

When you look at the ten major stressors listed in the above paragraphs, it becomes apparent that the possibility of stress can be found in nearly every aspect of our life. Sometimes, our lives get overwhelmed and we get anxious about managing things so that we have enough time for everything yet your commitments and responsibilities should not cause the feeling of stress that takes over our lives or begins to affect the overall physical and mental well-being.

How do you tell when you've reached the limit?

The signs of stress

In addition, keeping the causes for stress, we should be aware of the negative consequences. Yes, there are evident signs that you are being stressed out! Some are psychological, however, the same can be physical. Let's look at the negatives that could result from the accumulation of stressors within your life, instead of managing them and decreasing the impact of them.

Frequent Headaches

A lack of flow of blood, tiredness or illness are typically the causes of headaches as well as the most severe type of migraines. The fast breathing that people usually display as a way to "keep in tune" with the mental tumult of stress could trigger headaches,

A Greater Need to cry

Crying is your body's way of "releasing" emotional tensions which aren't addressed in a conscious way. That is when you're too distracted to address the natural emotions of sadness, anger or anxiety then your body will eventually try to release some of the trapped energy.

Unintentional weight gain or loss

Stress can have two different consequences on our appetites. you either are too overwhelmed in our thoughts about eating, or to be hungry, which leads us to not consume food, or we start to believe that we require more food to keep pace with the energy we're using which leads us to eat more. It is happening without even conscious of it or even noticing it.

Digestive Problems

Digestive disorders are among the most frequently reported symptoms of stress. The bowels and the intestines are affected by stress, absence of sleep, a changes in eating habits, or simply due to how exhausted an individual's body is when it is working for too long and putting in a lot of energy.

Anxiety and panic attacks

It is the body's way of signalling to us that we're juggling too many responsibilities and overloading ourselves. Stress and anxiety are the normal response of the body when we do not address our problems or fail to manage stress. This is extremely difficult to manage in the course of the day.

Inability to fall asleep or stay Sleepy

The stress of life can cause your brain to be racing, and when the brain is trying in order to cope with your thoughts plans, expectations, and plans it can be impossible to slow down. Like the principle that if you workout prior to bed, your body will be full of energy, and it will be harder to getting to sleep, working out your mind can also keep your body from sleeping.

Irritability Increasing

Stress can be a source of frustration. Feeling frustrated due to stress can lead to emotions that fluctuate, such as increased anger and paranoia, as well as overreaction and general being annoyed. This can lead to difficulties at workplace, at home, or in close relationships when yelling or withdrawing can occur.

Do you think you're dealing with a moderate level of anxiety in your daily life, or do you believe you're on the limit of "too too much?" If you consider yourself to be at a minimum stressed, and you're displaying any of the symptoms mentioned It could be time to think about whether the source of your issue is the level of stress that you're enduring.

Chapter 11: Controlling The Cravings, And Addictions

Human beings are extremely vulnerable to addiction. Collectively, we have always been and will likely always be. There's something unique about us how we're wired, our body's chemistry as well as the things we love and dislike, as well as our habits that we acquire throughout our lives that makes us human beings in general vulnerable to certain opportunities that are available throughout the world. These temptations aren't the same for everyone of us. Some are alcoholics but others are able to drink alcohol without issue. Some individuals have a problem with smoking, and others have found the determination to end their addiction forever. There are those who suffer from addictions that manifest in a particular social setting like an addiction to outrage. Some are also dependent on work.

Addictions can come in all forms and sizes, but what they all have in common is their negative, overwhelming impact upon our daily lives. Many of us have experienced what it is like to be affected by an addiction, whether due to the fact that we've been through one during the past, or in the present, or maybe because we've watched someone close to us, a family member or loved one fight against the monsters of addiction.

If it's an obsession with sugary food or crack cocaine or crack cocaine, the thoughts, emotions and actions that addictions can cause in our brains and bodies are identical.

My curiosity about using EFT tapping to treat for addictions stems from my experiences and studies into the use of EFT tapping to overcome the craving for food items. When I was researching the subject about weight loss I frequently meet people who held the mindset of weight loss being simple. "Just quit eating!" they'd say as if the words were the answer to everyone struggling with weight. I've heard the exact statement regarding alcoholics. "Just quit drinking!"

However, the reality is that a decision by itself is not enough and anyone who has had to deal with an issue with weight or addiction to alcohol recognizes that. The reason that they're not effective is because there is much more happening "behind those scenes" that can be the cause of our uncontrollable cravings. The good-hearted people who shout at the addict to stop their destructive behavior could just as well be shouting at a ball bouncing down a slope or a rock that falls off an rock. They could shout "stop" at any volume and often as they wish however it will not end anything in the least.

When I began digging into these subjects following my recovery from them, the common cause to all of the addictions was apparent. Alcohol, smoking and eating, consuming or procrastination, you know it all. They are all "escapism". This is our attempt, sometimes unconscious, to avoid having to deal with something that we're not used to, do not like or fear. We'll do whatever it takes to get rid of what is bothering us and drives us into the darkness of addiction.

If a thought, or a feeling an idea, pops up in your head when you're trying to pay attention to something other than that, do you let distract you? Perhaps, sometimes but most of the time, you do not. The distraction is put away or to somewhere in the background of your mind and concentrate on the task at hand. Everyone has a basic method of doing this that we've learned over the years. The basic mechanism we come up with without testing isn't a perfect one. This is why we can become so distracted that we forget about the work we're doing. The mechanism is not without limits and those limits establish the point at which your internal power ceases and is replaced by external power source.

This external power could be in the form of someone speaking to you in a way that can triggers emotions and distracts you from thinking. It could be the shape or bad news positive news, an odor or sight that has importance,

134

or even another thing entirely. However, whatever it is and in whatever way you're unable to handle it, you're left powerless in the presence of something larger than you. If you lose the ability to control your own life that you naturally are endowed with, and that lack of control creates an adverse impact on your life, it could be suffering from an addiction.

In our heads there are programs running constantly, just like programs on computers. They could be thought of as films, images and slide show. It is not uncommon for memories to move through our minds whether in the front or in the background. It is especially evident when we're trying to sleep. For the majority of us we don't have a clear idea of what is causing this, or how to stop it. It is likely that you don't know how to alter the images of "movies" that play on your mind at any given moment like the majority of people aren't sure how to manage their addictions.

We all share the same in the sense that we're all in control of some thing. The limitations of our authority and control over ourselves are what set us apart. In this regard the self-control we exercise and willpower, self-control, and ultimately our ability to overcome habits that drag us down is similar to muscles. If not trained it will be tinier and weak. Our power-spread and control over us will be a tiny one too. However, as we do the difficult but rewarding work of building that muscle our control expands and grows until we look at the things that made us powerless in the past and understand that they're nothing to us today. We can defeat them, because we are strong and more powerful than their negative influence over us. This is the meaning to defeat addiction.

Reconnecting painful past memories

To be ready to conquer your addictions requires being prepared to confront those things that been a source of pain through the years. You must confront them first , and secondly, you have to do your best to transform the way you deal with them. It's not easy. It's much easier to keep doing the same thing. It's easier to continue smoking, drinking, shouting eating, or whatever other harmful behaviors our lifestyles require us to engage in. We would all prefer to stick with the routine instead of confronting the trauma and agony of our experiences in the past. We're taught to think and act in these ways without even contemplating the consequences. When you hear a specific item, or in a specific situation which triggers something within you, like the smell of an alcohol advertisement or the scent of cigarettes or the smell of a cigarette, we're stimulated like Pavlov's dog, losing control of our minds, and focusing on what's likely to be the next thing.

Within us we are able to record memories through our entire lives. The memories we have, an enormous degree, determine our thoughts, emotions, and our actions throughout the day. Let me provide you with an illustration of what I'm speaking about. When I was around 10 years old, I recall getting involved in a schoolyard battle. Some other kids joined in on me and attempted to beat me. I was terrified and fled away from them but they retreated on me, and they beat me up with a branch of the tree. It was a terrifying and painful experience for me at the time and for some time following. However, when I share this story now it is no longer affecting me emotionally. It was for a while but not today. It's not because, If I allow it to happen go, who's beat me today with a stick? It's not the 10 year old boys on the playground. It's me. I'm just getting myself into a bind whenever I think about this past memory and let it dictate any of my actions, thoughts or emotions at the moment.

In my analogy in the past about "movies" being played out in our minds and this is what I'm referring to. There's a movie about me getting separated and going through the middle of a divorce that is very painful, however, it's just an actual film. It's not just an actual movie and I am the director of the movie. I control it, and not the opposite. In addition, however much memories can be able to control us, memories aren't actual things. They are just memories. The actual events took place sometime in the distant past. perhaps the far distant past. There's no reason to the control of our memories that we have experienced. our lives. We can separate them from our thinking and actions in the present, and let them be. They might always be present within our minds but they don't always control our actions.

I've worked hard to overcome my addictions, and to separate those painful experiences from motive that drives my actions in my current-day life. There is no distinction between me and you. I'm not smarter or better, or more special or special in any manner. The only difference is that

I've learned the strategies that will help you conquer the urges to drink and other addictions one for all. When you learn and master this technique and techniques, you will also be able to achieve the similar inner power.

The connection between memories and Addictions

I'd like to ensure I have the time to clarify why memories are crucial when it comes to addiction. Many times, people don't realize the link between addiction and memory. They don't get much help from the standard medical establishment's view of addictions as a result of chemical issues that is usually treated with (surprise!) prescription drugs. In certain situations this may work however my experience and research suggest that, in the majority of cases there's a better method.

The reason memory is significant is that they account for the blocks that are present within usthat hinder the flow of energy throughout our bodies. When energy doesn't flow as it is supposed to it should, we lose our natural balance. We find ourselves increasingly disengaged from our goals and things that make us feel happy and healthy. It is possible to accomplish certain things but we'll never realize our full potential. Like a tree, if it has to be grown near to the wall that is a brick structure the roots of the tree will be affected, and its growth will be slowed. It could still grow to an impressive size and strength, but it will be weaker and smaller than it would have been without the wall in front of it.

EFT tapping can be the most simple, most efficient, and effective method I've ever encountered for breaking down the "walls" which are preventing our growth and restricting our possibilities.

When we tap the blockages with an appropriate tapping program, we are able to work on removing the blockage, eventually removing it completely and restoring the energy flow our bodies are designed to experience. Self-esteem, willpower and the ability to change our negative habits are all derived from the person we are in our real self. We do not come with addictions. They become result of our daily experiences and the blocks they create. EFT tapping provides the technique that lets us turn back the time of addiction to a past time before the energy that flows naturally through the body was diminished and to a time where we weren't an inmate within the prison of addiction.

Utilizing EFT tapping to help with addiction recovery

Through tapping into our destructive memories and current addictions We can start to alter the way we think about these experiences as well as their impact on us in the present and into the future. We cannot alter the exact moment that took place in the first place, but that is not in the present, and it's set in the stone. But it doesn't matter. What's important to us in the future is how we will remember it.

Always, prior to you start tapping, take a few minutes to tune into your body. On a scale from 1 to 10, you can gauge the level of discomfort that your addiction currently causing you. While you work through your addiction, remember that you're in charge in this situation. This is your energy and is only yours to you.

Tapping Process

Begin by tapping your fingers four times on the point one. the hand's side (or"karate chop" point) "karate chop" point). Tap lightly. There's no reason to be angry with yourself or cause harm to yourself. Speak out loudly:

"Even although I feel I am getting out of control at the moment I deeply and completely embrace and accept myself. I deeply love and accept how I am feeling right now. I am deeply grateful and love myself and all that I am."

Continue to tap on the second point of your wrist's inner part. Tap with your fingers with two or four or with your other wrist. Speak loudly:

"Even although I feel ashamed and sadness about my addiction and my inability to manage it. Although I often believe that I will never be hooked. Although I sometimes believe I am unable to overcome this addiction , because I'm weak, and it's too powerful. Although I may feel that way I deeply respect and love me, my body and my mind, as well as how I am feeling right now."

The next step is tapping the third point, at the high point on your head. Tap all four fingers of both hands, and then say loudly:

"I enjoy the way that my body feels this moment. I am sure that my body will do the most beneficial for me. My mind desires the most beneficial for me. I am aware that my feelings of sadness and shame regarding my addiction are my body's way of

146

ensuring that I am paying focus on my overall health and wellbeing. I accept and love that my body is trying to tell me to be secure from danger. I am deeply thankful for this response. I cherish and embrace all parts of my body. I am grateful for everything it can do for me."

Continue to tap the fourth point, your eyebrows. You can tap one side using two fingers. Switch sides after going through the tapping process again. Speak loudly as you tap:

"I know what it is like to conquer my fears. It's a thrill to accomplish things I thought I could not do. I've felt what it's like to accomplish the goals I made for myself. I accept and love the fact that my body needs to end this addiction. Although I feel feeling of shame and discontent in myself for having allowed my addiction to spiral beyond control I'm aware of what my ultimate success will look and look like."

Continue to tap the fifth point on the part of the eye that is on your side. Tap your fingers with two fingers either side. After you have completed the tapping sequence a third time, it is possible to are able to switch sides. As you tap:

"I am determined to get well and healthy once more. Able to be free of addiction as I was meant to be. I see myself moving past my blocks and difficulties and releasing myself from the regret and displeasure of addiction. I am confident that I can do it. I am confident that I can restore my body's natural peace and energy flow."

Continue to tap at the 6th point, underneath your eyes. Tap two fingers either side. If you repeat the same tapping sequence the third time, it is possible to may switch sides. As you tap:

"I am in control of my body. I control my emotions. I am in control of all my feelings. I am in control of the flow of my energy. I am in charge and nobody else is able to take me under their control. I feel the power rising in me. I know that I am more powerful over this habit. I am confident without a shadow of doubt that I will beat this. I am able to feel my energy beginning to flow, as the blocks and disruptions get smaller."

Then, move to tapping the 7th point underneath your nose. Tap two fingers, and shout out loud while you tap:

"This ongoing shame and displeasure about my addiction is difficult for me to release. I know that my body doesn't wish to see me let go. I know that my body's desire to protect me. I am aware of and appreciative of all the things my body is doing for me. But I've also spent a lot of time thinking that I could not achieve it. I thought I could not overcome the addiction and lead an enlightened life."

Continue to tap the point 8 of your cheeks. Tap your fingers with two fingers. shout out loud while you tap:

"But I now love and accept that my body reacts in this manner. I deeply love and accept myself, despite this addiction, and all the pain and shame it brought into my life. I deeply love and accept each and every part of me, and I am confident that I'm capable of making my own decisions. I am confident that the acceptance and love I feel for myself will provide me with the courage I need to overcome that addiction."

The next step is tapping the collarbone at point 9. Tap on one side using your four fingers. Switch sides as you go through the tapping sequence a second time. As you tap:

"I am willing to give up this need to indulge in destructive behaviors. I don't need the negativity that I have in my life any longer. My strength is strong, and can live an addiction-free lifestyle. I feel the disappointment and guilt disappearing from my body. I feel the strength and determination to improve my health and well-being rising up within me. I have experienced this feeling of determination. I've experienced what it feels like to reach my goals. I've felt what it's to be able to face my fears and I feel these emotions inside me right now."

Then, move to tapping the point 10 beneath your arms. Tap the opposite side using the entire four fingers. Switch sides as you go through the tapping process the second time. As you tap:

Chapter 12: Resolve The Problem Of Addictions

Addiction can take many types - smoking, drugs or sex, shopping, food, etc. If you believe that you're not able to manage your habits and addictions to an extent that it impacts your health, you must seek the advice of a professional medical counsellor. EFT has helped many overcome addictions, and I'm sure it will assist you too. Research has proven that if you do the same thing for a period of 30-days, this can become a habit. Once a new habit has been developed, your brain creates an endocrine pathway, making the newly adopted habit easy to adhere to. It's important to be aware of this as it's possible to eliminate undesirable habits and develop new ones. The brain is able to adapt to some degree of plasticity to it. It is true that addiction isn't so simple as bad habits and good ones However, by getting rid of certain unhealthy habits and replacing them with healthier ones, you can help you overcome addiction more easily.

The limbic system of the brain produces chemical like serotonin and dopamine. Dopamine can trigger feelings such as "I should have this" when you look at an attractive outfit or nice car. Dopamine is a pleasure chemical that rewards certain behaviors regardless whether or not the activities are healthful. Consuming junk food releases dopamine, which can make it an enjoyable sensation, which increases the probability that you'll eat the junk food in order to experience the dopamine boost.

Serotonin is also a "feel well" chemical that is similar to dopamine. If your levels of serotonin are low, you're more likely to experience depression, addiction, etc. Through the practice of EFT and tapping, you'll be able overcome your addictions. The method using EFT taps releases serotonin that, produces an enjoyable feeling. This can help you avoid engaging in other enjoyable activities such as eating unhealthy food or smoking cigarettes. It is recommended to be doing your EFT as well as tapping on a regular basis and at specific times throughout the day. One example of a strategic time could be when you're exhausted at home after work , when you normally eat comfort food or prior to an evening out with your buddies to stay clear of drinking. Perform the EFT practice just prior to those moments when you're typically driven to get into the habit; this can help you replace your bad habit with a positive one.

Quitting smoking

Smoking cigarettes can cause lung cancer, a chronic illness. Smoking is not just detrimental to the health of you but also those close to you. Many smokers are aware that smoking is not a good choice, but they find it difficult to stop regardless of the dangers. Many tried to quit smoking cigarettes, but the withdrawal process was too hard for them, and they blinked. They suffered from "shakes" and the anxiety. Many people claim that they don't know what they should accomplish with the hands when they have cigarettes in them. This is usually a result of bad habits that were taught by smokers, and the good thing is that through EFT we can reverse the negative energy that has been created and establish the new positive and healthy pattern of behavior that can aid you in overcoming the addiction.

If you are suffering from withdrawal symptoms, your scripts for setting up your taps could include something like "Even even though I feel weak whenever I quit smoking I'm confident that this won't persist and that I'll eventually get over the smoking addiction".

Imagine that you're experiencing stress and you're unable to light an cigarette. How do you feel? If you experience uncomfortable in the stomach then you may be required to tap the outside of your stomach and declare "Even even though I am feeling a little uncomfortable in my stomach over quitting smoking, I'm sure the discomfort will ease and I am completely comfortable with my own feelings".

It's important to imagine how much better your life will be if you quit smoking cigarettes. Imagine how healthier you'd be, how well financially and how you wouldn't be one of the people who smoke outside while everybody else enjoys the warmth inside. If you find that this positive image isn't effective enough for you, then it might be better to try the opposite. Make a picture that you can visualize in your head of the way your life could get worse due to the smoking habits you have. What will it be the experience for your friends and family members if they had to come visit you in a hospital due to lung cancer? It's an excellent illustration, but you must be able to develop the vision that you desire in your head that is powerful enough to spur you to stopping for the good.

A few of the tapping setup scripts could be utilized include: (Again, it depends on the situation, and you can modify it to suit your needs.)

A) "Even although I smoke to manage anxiety, I am completely comfortable with my own health and will look for better options to deal with stress".

B) "Even even though I only smoke when I'm with my family, I still be a loving person to my family and myself and not smoke".

C) "Even even though I feel guilty for this addiction issue, I fully embrace and love myself".

Click here to view an instructional video on how to use EFT to quit smoking.

Quitting Alcohol

Drinking excessively puts your health in danger and can cause a variety of health-related problems, such as liver disease and high blood pressure osteoporosis and heart disease and even issues with fertility. A few drinks while you're at a party is not a sign that you are an alcohol addict. But, when it starts to dominate all of the time and becomes a hindrance to your daily life and negatively impacts your relationships and work, the time is now to alter your lifestyle. If you experience shakes or anxiety after not drinking for a couple of days then you should consider using EFT or tapping in order to aid deal withdrawal symptoms. It is highly advised to consult an expert regarding this issue.

To combat this addiction, just like other addictions, it is necessary to determine the root causes of the addiction. If you can identify the root of the problem and becoming aware of it , the more control you will have over it. If you are aware of factors like stress, loneliness or social situations that lead to the drinking that you do, then you are able to intervene and put yourself on the back foot before going down the slippery slope. Try to come up with a healthier alternative for these triggers that could assist you in getting rid of your addiction to alcohol. Naturally, using techniques such as EFT and tapping can assist you.

EFT tapping scripts to treat alcohol dependence

Make sure you follow the 5 steps in chapter 5 while using the tapping scripts below:

"Even although I am nervous when I don't drink alcohol, I'm sure that this anxiety will fade and I'll eventually break that habit".

"Even although I've always been an alcoholic I have accepted and cherish myself to the fullest, and am determined to overcome this habit".

"Even although I drink as my father did I am adamant and devoted to myself unconditionally and have learned the right habits, too".

"Even even though I drink to combat my solitude, I forgive myself and am in love with myself".

Eating disorders

Emotional eating is a typical eating disorder, and could lead to unintentional and unhealthy weight increase. Patients suffering from this condition eat to relax themselves or simply out of routine. It's not the person's blame, but it's something they can correct. For certain people, eating junk food, especially unhealthy food, can release a number of feel-good chemicals in the brain such as serotonin and dopamine. It's these chemicals that cause people to crave food every time they're feeling low.

If you are eating because you're unhappy, sad, or depressed or you're craving sugary food items such as sugar or chocolate,, then tapping and EFT can aid you. It's about removing this negative energy and replace it with a positive one.

EFT is a method to manage eating disorders

It is important to adhere to the five steps when using the setup scripts below and be sure to rate your craving between 1 and 10 prior to and after you've completed the tapping sequence and the script. Here are some instances of tap scripts that can be used for eating disorders. However, please be sure to modify the script to suit your needs. If for instance you discover yourself eating excessively due to an unresolved breakup You should add this to your customized setting script.

Chapter 13: Tapping And Shivershaking(Tm)

When you stand, lift your heels in alternating ways off the ground , and then accelerate it until that your entire body starts to shiver.

Each time take note of how it vibrates the entire body. Then, gently put fingers on the face, and then feel the vibrating. This will increase the vital microcirculation of your face.

However, I would suggest that you place your right wrist ahead of your left hand, so that your left wrist is close to the body. This triggers the nerves that feed your eyes, so you are able to see better.

Wart Reduction

The wart of this woman was reduced dramatically through the use of these techniques in a series of phases, over several weeks.

"I was plagued by a large small wart in my right hand. it was very tender and painful. I was determined to get it removed however, I wanted also to address the root cause, as I had observed that it was likely to develop again using different ways.

Through the use of techniques to get rid of the virus and improve circulation to the affected area the infection gradually faded away and hasn't returned since. I'm also certain that I'm healthier as due to the exercise I'm doing every day to maintain my skin's health."

I recommend to Shivershake(tm) in each Hand Position to achieve the optimal results.

We all recognize that if you adhere to the advice of your teacher or read this book carefully and enjoy a lot of laughs the body will be activated. face as well as various body organs to firm and allow your visible wrinkles to diminish. In the end, due to the toxicity that is held within your cells, gravity of the earth and poor habits your face will begin to fall and then become more saggy and spongy.

However the Face Lift Yoga(tm) is the answer to this! It is possible to maintain and enhance your lifting at home every day, wearing the Cleopatra skin Face Lift Headband! It only takes half an hour per day or one minute every day if you take the Accelerated Pampering Technique(tm) during your Advanced Class or Cleopatra Skin Face Lift Yoga classes.

The neck and shoulders can be stiff prior to ... then after about 30 minutes. You can achieve useful, effective results by mudras, breathing and Everlasting Creams(tm) when you can hold them long enough with Everlasting Pots(tm).

Accelerated Rejuvenation

In the blink of an eye, the 87-year-old man got up from his bed and broke the right leg of his femur. He underwent surgery and a pin placed inside the bone. Following that, he was put on an array of medications that did not stop him from being free of extreme pain.

In reality, the only thing he experienced that provided him with significant relief from pain was massage. However, his daughter who was the one who managed his money of which he was a king, would not pay for massages or take massages as a present from friends. Therefore, he was still in the pain and was deluded by his medication.

The doctor gave him three weeks of life by the medical professionals He took the decision to adopt the natural health regimen practiced by his son who took him from care in a nursing facility and put him into private home care. Within three weeks, he had been completely off of any medication and his blood pressure was at a normal level after the first time for years and his delusions were gone and his pain levels were lower.

The result was that within two months, he no longer felt pain and was able to walk around the house with no stick or walker. Even though the five times he fell and had to be rescued, he was not injured or injuries and could stand up with only a little help.

Significantly, his ability to think increased dramatically. He was a champion in chess, and had drawn an international champion in 1934. After that, was back to playing great chess.

He was a fan of exercising for an hour at the pool each day, and massages to relax him every three days.

The result was astonishing. In the following six months, with dramatically improved quality of living the man was at peace dying, and he left his body in peace.

"My dad, Jo who fell down, injured the right leg of his. In the following year, there was a lot of pain throughout his hips, right leg, and back. At the age of 87, Jo suffered from constant and severe pain. Jo's life had become "hell". He was suffering from 110 different ailments and was given three weeks to live by his physician.

After two months of natural therapy, Jo was free of pain and was completely off all his medication and walking independently. It was a combination of Shivershaking(tm) along with Superstretching(tm) to ease back pain, particularly at night when he was waking up with discomfort. In some instances, he'd have to repeat this process several times a night, from any comfy posture, but it was effective and eventually he experienced full back pain relief as well as sleeping well regularly." Don More, Back Pain Relief Association

"This woman suffered from extreme back pain. Scoliosis which is a the spine is twisted - prior to ... as well also after two days. The patient had rods put through her spinal canal (see the scars down to the back of her lower) and was in pain following that procedure. Therefore, she had the rods removed. She then attended one of our workshops and provided herself as a demonstration model. The back pain went away within ten minutes and her spine was straightened within two days. The spine was not straight however. In order to achieve this, she had follow the complete schedule for about 4 to 5 months. After that, she had her own face Lift!" D R More.

"I was diagnosed with Scheuermann's disease which is a genetic disorder in the spinal. I attended a workshop over the weekend organized through the Back Pain Relief Association, and returned home.

In front of the mirror I took a 'before picture of the curve on my upper back in my usual posture. Then I followed the method that was taught in the class over seven minutes. After that, I took the "after photo, with what appeared to be my not-so-great posture. I had strayed a bit.

Also, I had the distinction of being a world champion Moto-Cross rider. I was injured by a fractured collar bone, as well as fractures to other bones, too. I learned to live with it', which included the discomfort and pain.

Then I've found the methods I require to eliminate the discomfort and pain and adjust my neck bone. My arms were weak to be able to ride on a motorbike, but after realigning my spine as well as other bones, they've been strengthened. I am able to ride my bike once more. I am very thankful for the many benefits that this has brought me." David Clothier, Australia

Rainbow Tapping(tm)

Vibration is the link between all things. When you generalize the impact of the vibration, it's not as powerful, but it is more delicate. The more specific you define it, the more focused and strong the impact on the area in question. You get fast results.

The perfectly-crafted affirmation, of the The Everlasting Cream "Feet heal quickly now" that is sung in a down-scale manner - which is from high to low and then tapping your feet, identifies the feet. If your feet hurt it could help quicker in comparison to "Whole body heals quickly".

The Chromatic Rainbow Charts

They will show you how to define one-twelfth of your body. It's a good start. Making use of your 12 Colorful Rainbow Reflexology Maps(tm) are much more precise and beneficial. Perform this procedure for every Color of the Chromatic Rainbow Colour.

Utilize other methods like music, colour, food, gemstones, essential oils, and other substances to increase the effects. They enhance the effect since they have more precise. One example is Nutgrass. It helps loosen the lower ribcage region and in particular, helps to sharpen flat voices and enhances in your singing voice, while giving it a vibrant look.

For best results, breathe abdominally with your Baby's Natural Tongue

Position, read the books and charts and listen to the music on www.FaceLiftYoga.com.Au

Each key in the musical serves a purpose, it has it has a healing effect. It activates Reflexology Maps and specific areas of your body, changing an unfavourable response into an optimistic.

The Brain is in Your Belly

There are three kinds of addictions. Head addictions are when you're obsessed with being right or wrong instead of just being practical and practical.

Heart addictions happen when you're dependent on feeling low or up instead of feeling healthy. You need the drama of your life to make you feel like you're living.

Belly addictions happen when you're addicted to being hungry or feeling full (comfort food) instead of just being full.

You have threeseparate nervous systems within your body that can be independent and operate in a way that is interdependent - your brain and the heart (sino-atrial node) and your stomach (enteric nervous system).

It is possible to Rainbow Tap to gain bliss throughout the entire body, stomach, heart, or head. As you experience more bliss, the amount of addiction decreases until you are no longer obsessed with thinking eating, feeling or taking drugs, and so on.

Each day, shake shivershake throughout the day while Rainbow tapping the three areas. The majority of your time will be spent on the part that displays the highest amount of dependence.

Be sure to breathe using the Baby's Natural Tongue position as tapping. Do you know that around the 80% of people who suffer from depression start to improve their emotional state by removing any metal from their bodies by breathing deeply in the Baby's Natural Tongue position as illustrated, and drinking pure water? If you breathe in, your belly, you should let it go.

Conclusion

The fast-paced lifestyle we live is not good for living a healthy, joyful life. We're always chasing a idea or another, and forgetting the things that matter to us the most. As a result, we're facing a life-threatening burnout. One of the best methods to fight burnout from work is to abandon your job and begin with a new career. Homework can protect your from the stress that a 9-to-5 job brings.

The first step to combat burnout is to get away off from working. This could be a brief vacation, taking advantage of your sick time or taking a short break from work so that you're free from the negative atmosphere. The time off can allow you to recharge and gain new perspectives on your life, career and the best path to follow.

Work from home is becoming more popular today. It is among the fastest-growing new business forms currently available. When you establish your business from home allows you to be flexible that isn't available when you rent or purchase out a warehouse or office space. Even if you work from home and requires discipline and discipline, the advantages you reap are huge.

Although it's the case that not all business models, specifically home-based companies, work well but the lower expenses involved can reduce the chance of losing money significantly. The greatest benefit you can get with a home office is that you have the opportunity to try out new ideas without the expense of cost. It will allow you to determine the feasibility of a specific company before investing a lot of money in it.

It is also possible to scale up or scale down depending on the results the company is experiencing. When you rent office, it is restricted by the size of the office, which means the process of scaling down or expanding is complicated to control. However, a home-based system allows you to work for less or extended hours and hire the right amount of people.

If you work at home, you have various flexibility and freedoms that allow you to grow your company at whatever speed you'd like. It is also possible to save money in a variety of different ways. This is important in the early phases of the business.

The most important benefit is that you're not confined by your work schedule, challenging boss or coworkers or the stress of your normal 9-to-5 job. It's about time to say goodbye to the stress-filled lifestyle and welcome the peace that comes with working from your home.